The Sickly Pumpkin's Chronic Health Handbook

L & R May

ISBN: 9781797794594

DEDICATION

This book is for everyone who has been ill and struggled to get a diagnosis or effective treatment, and for everyone supporting somebody with chronic ill health.

CONTENTS

ACKNOWLEDGMENTS

With thanks to all the people who offered help and suggestions when we were both ill, to our local EDS support group and to everyone who helped us to improve this handbook and make it the most useful it could possibly be.

1 INTRODUCTION

In an ideal world, you'd notice something not quite right, make an appointment and see a doctor, who would diagnose you and offer treatment.

This might work well for 'obvious' ailments, but there are a lot of people with more complex problems who struggle to get diagnosed because their symptoms vary over time, or their local GP is not familiar with their rare illness.

We're both very familiar with the frustration of repeatedly going to the doctor for a short consultation where they don't have time to understand your history, and leaving no further along, or with medication which treats your symptoms and not the underlying causes.

Even when the doctor refers you to a specialist, the process can often be confusing and you might struggle to remember crucial information when they ask you, or to understand the relevance of their questions.

If you're admitted to hospital, it's helpful for the staff to have access to detailed information about your condition and medical history.

This little book is designed to support you through your medical journey – it's a place for you to make a note of all your symptoms and the different things you've tried, all the people you've spoken to and the conclusions they've drawn. We hope that it will help you to get a diagnosis, and at the very least it will help you learn how to manage your illness so that you suffer less and don't accidentally trigger it.

We also hope that this book will be helpful in demonstrating the effects of your illness to officials if you need to claim benefits, or ask for special help at work.

When we were trying to get diagnosed with our own conditions, we found that we got the best results by presenting our symptoms to the doctor in an orderly way – we found ourselves writing timelines, drawing graphs, lists of bullet points – any way we could think of to communicate what we were experiencing in a way that they could use to help us. We have put all of these tools together and tested them with other patients.

Please use as much of this book, or as little, as you want. There are plenty of blank pages for your own notes, and so that you can staple in appointment cards and letters.

We hope that it helps you, or the person you are caring for. If you think of other tools we could include, please let us know!

- Lillith & Rebecca May

2 ABOUT ME

The key information that your medical providers will need to know..

Name	
Date of Birth	
Address	
Telephone number(s)	
Email address(es)	
Emergency Contact(s)	

Doctor's Surgery address, GP and telephone number

Social worker, Care worker, Advocate etc

NHS Number

Allergies

Current diagnosed chronic illnesses:

Effects of current illnesses on other treatments (i.e. Physiotherapy, Anaesthesitics, etc):

Work (Any physical/visual/mental requirements or risks)

Caring duties and responsibilities (People and pets!)

Dietary Requirements

Have you had any aids and adaptations to your house, for example wet rooms or wheelchair access? Is this something you might need in the future?

Other:

3 MEDICAL HISTORY & TEST RESULTS

Fill out as much as you can remember..

PLACE OF BIRTH:
BLOOD TYPE:
CHILDHOOD ILLNESSES:
HOSPITAL VISITS:

IMMUNISATIONS:

IMMUNISATIONS:

OPERATIONS:

OUTPATIENT TREATMENTS:

BROKEN BONES/TRAUMATIC INJURIES?

LONG TERM PHYSICAL DISABILITIES:

OTHER CHRONIC ISSUES: (i.e. Gastric, Menstrual, Mental Health, Heart, Lungs etc)

TEST RESULTS

DATE:

TEST (Blood, Urine, Scan etc)

REQUESTED BY (Medical professional)

TESTED BY: (Lab etc)

TESTING FOR:

RESULTS:

NOTES:

DATE:

TEST (Blood, Urine, Scan etc)

REQUESTED BY (Medical professional)

TESTED BY: (Lab etc)

TESTING FOR:

RESULTS:

NOTES:

DATE:

TEST (Blood, Urine, Scan etc)

REQUESTED BY (Medical professional)

TESTED BY: (Lab etc)

TESTING FOR:

RESULTS:

NOTES:

DATE:

TEST (Blood, Urine, Scan etc)

REQUESTED BY (Medical professional)

TESTED BY: (Lab etc)

TESTING FOR:

RESULTS:

NOTES:

DATE:

TEST (Blood, Urine, Scan etc)

REQUESTED BY (Medical professional)

TESTED BY: (Lab etc)

TESTING FOR:

RESULTS:

NOTES:

DATE:

TEST (Blood, Urine, Scan etc)

REQUESTED BY (Medical professional)

TESTED BY: (Lab etc)

TESTING FOR:

RESULTS:

NOTES:

DATE:

TEST (Blood, Urine, Scan etc)

REQUESTED BY (Medical professional)

TESTED BY: (Lab etc)

TESTING FOR:

RESULTS:

NOTES:

DATE:

TEST (Blood, Urine, Scan etc)

REQUESTED BY (Medical professional)

TESTED BY: (Lab etc)

TESTING FOR:

RESULTS:

NOTES:

DATE:

TEST (Blood, Urine, Scan etc)

REQUESTED BY (Medical professional)

TESTED BY: (Lab etc)

TESTING FOR:

RESULTS:

NOTES:

DATE:

TEST (Blood, Urine, Scan etc)

REQUESTED BY (Medical professional)

TESTED BY: (Lab etc)

TESTING FOR:

RESULTS:

NOTES:

4 FAMILY HISTORY

Lots of illnesses and allergies run in families. It can be helpful to ask your immediate family about any ailments they suffer from; it can often make diagnosis much quicker.

MOTHER

FATHER

FATHER

SIBLINGS AND HALF SIBLINGS

23

GRANDPARENTS (MATERNAL)

SIBLINGS AND HALF SIBLINGS

GRANDPARENTS (PATERNAL)

CHILDREN

COUSINS

OTHER

5 MEDICATIONS

Here's a place for you to list all the medications you have been prescribed.

Name of medication
Dose
Date started taking
Date finished taking
What was the medication for?
Did you have any side effects?
What lifestyle changes do you have to make for the medication to work effectively? (i.e. no alcohol etc)
Notes

Medication
Dose
Date started taking
Date finished taking
What was the medication for?
Side effects
Lifestyle changes
Notes

Medication
Dose
Date started taking
Date finished taking
What was the medication for?
Side effects
Lifestyle changes
Notes

Medication
Dose
Date started taking
Date finished taking
What was the medication for?
Side effects
Lifestyle changes
Notes

Medication
Dose
Date started taking
Date finished taking
What was the medication for?
Side effects
Lifestyle changes
Notes

Medication
Dose
Date started taking
Date finished taking
What was the medication for?
Side effects
Lifestyle changes
Notes

Medication
Dose
Date started taking
Date finished taking
What was the medication for?
Side effects
Lifestyle changes
Notes

Medication
Dose
Date started taking
Date finished taking
What was the medication for?
Side effects
Lifestyle changes
Notes

Medication
Dose
Date started taking
Date finished taking
What was the medication for?
Side effects
Lifestyle changes
Notes

Medication
Dose
Date started taking
Date finished taking
What was the medication for?
Side effects
Lifestyle changes
Notes

Medication
Dose
Date started taking
Date finished taking
What was the medication for?
Side effects
Lifestyle changes
Notes

Medication
Dose
Date started taking
Date finished taking
What was the medication for?
Side effects
Lifestyle changes
Notes

Medication
Dose
Date started taking
Date finished taking
What was the medication for?
Side effects
Lifestyle changes
Notes

Medication
Dose
Date started taking
Date finished taking
What was the medication for?
Side effects
Lifestyle changes
Notes

Medication
Dose
Date started taking
Date finished taking
What was the medication for?
Side effects
Lifestyle changes
Notes

Medication
Dose
Date started taking
Date finished taking
What was the medication for?
Side effects
Lifestyle changes
Notes

Medication
Dose
Date started taking
Date finished taking
What was the medication for?
Side effects
Lifestyle changes
Notes

Medication
Dose
Date started taking
Date finished taking
What was the medication for?
Side effects
Lifestyle changes
Notes

Medication
Dose
Date started taking
Date finished taking
What was the medication for?
Side effects
Lifestyle changes
Notes

Medication
Dose
Date started taking
Date finished taking
What was the medication for?
Side effects
Lifestyle changes
Notes

Medication
Dose
Date started taking
Date finished taking
What was the medication for?
Side effects
Lifestyle changes
Notes

Medication
Dose
Date started taking
Date finished taking
What was the medication for?
Side effects
Lifestyle changes
Notes

Medication
Dose
Date started taking
Date finished taking
What was the medication for?
Side effects
Lifestyle changes
Notes

Medication
Dose
Date started taking
Date finished taking
What was the medication for?
Side effects
Lifestyle changes
Notes

Medication
Dose
Date started taking
Date finished taking
What was the medication for?
Side effects
Lifestyle changes
Notes

6 DIAGNOSES

Fill in this section whenever a medical professional confirms a diagnosis with you.

<table>
<tr><td>What was diagnosed?</td></tr>
<tr><td>When?</td></tr>
<tr><td>By which doctor? (Contact details if possible)/Attach a copy of the letter</td></tr>
<tr><td>What effects will the illness have on you?</td></tr>
<tr><td>What lifestyle changes were recommended?</td></tr>
<tr><td>What treatment was recommended?</td></tr>
<tr><td>Are you being referred to another specialist?</td></tr>
</table>

Sickly Pumpkin's Chronic Health Handbook

<table>
<tr><td>

What was diagnosed?

43

</td></tr>
<tr><td>

When?

</td></tr>
<tr><td>

By which doctor? (Contact details if possible)/Attach a copy of the letter

</td></tr>
<tr><td>

What effects will the illness have on you?

</td></tr>
<tr><td>

What lifestyle changes were recommended?

</td></tr>
<tr><td>

What treatment was recommended?

</td></tr>
<tr><td>

Are you being referred to another specialist?

</td></tr>
</table>

44

What was diagnosed?
When?
By which doctor? (Contact details if possible)/Attach a copy of the letter
What effects will the illness have on you?
What lifestyle changes were recommended?
What treatment was recommended?
Are you being referred to another specialist?

What was diagnosed?
When?
By which doctor? (Contact details if possible)/Attach a copy of the letter
What effects will the illness have on you?
What lifestyle changes were recommended?
What treatment was recommended?
Are you being referred to another specialist?

What was diagnosed?
When?
By which doctor? (Contact details if possible)/Attach a copy of the letter
What effects will the illness have on you?
What lifestyle changes were recommended?
What treatment was recommended?
Are you being referred to another specialist?

Sickly Pumpkin's Chronic Health Handbook

What was diagnosed?
When?
By which doctor? (Contact details if possible)/Attach a copy of the letter
What effects will the illness have on you?
What lifestyle changes were recommended?
What treatment was recommended?
Are you being referred to another specialist?

What was diagnosed?
When?
By which doctor? (Contact details if possible)/Attach a copy of the letter
What effects will the illness have on you?
What lifestyle changes were recommended?
What treatment was recommended?
Are you being referred to another specialist?

What was diagnosed?
When?
By which doctor? (Contact details if possible)/Attach a copy of the letter
What effects will the illness have on you?
What lifestyle changes were recommended?
What treatment was recommended?
Are you being referred to another specialist?

7 SYMPTOMS

It can be difficult to assess your symptoms as they can change over time and be masked by lifestyle changes or other illnesses.

Further on in the book we'll provide a daily diary for you to use ; this space is for recording any long term symptoms that you've suffered from.

It can be helpful to do this on a timeline, for example:

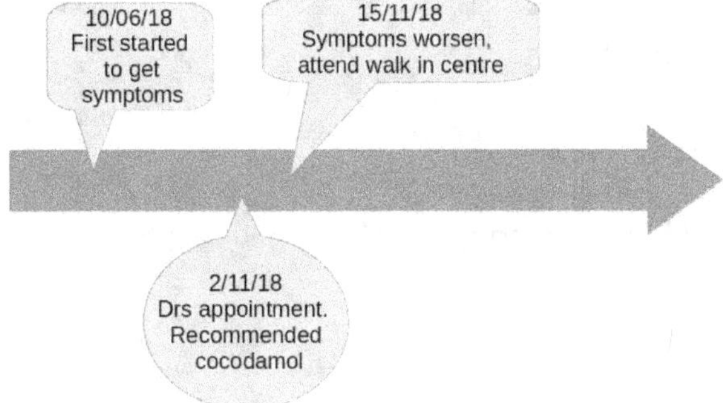

It can also be helpful to show them on a diagram.

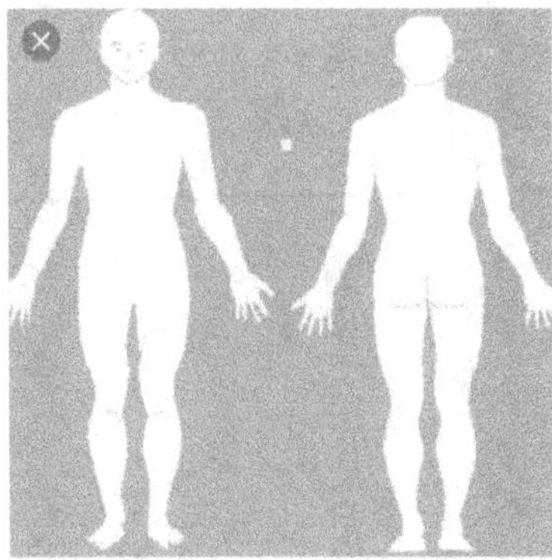

Date
Symptom
Severity
How is this affecting you?
Any ideas what might have caused it?
How are you treating it?
Did you speak to a medical professional or pharmacist and what was the outcome?
Have you had this before?

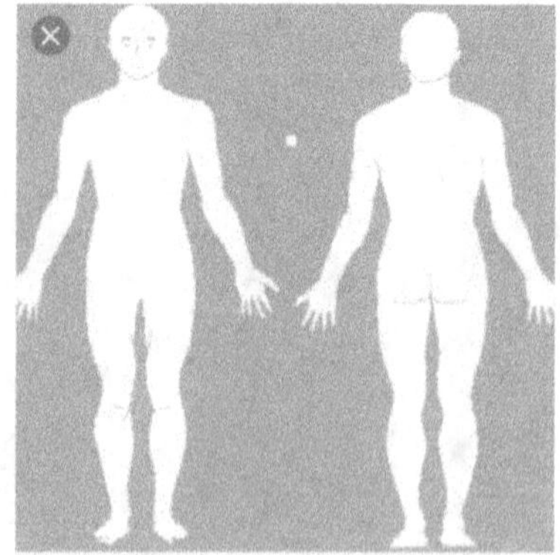

Date
Symptom
Severity
How is this affecting you?
Any ideas what might have caused it?
How are you treating it?
Did you speak to a medical professional or pharmacist and what was the outcome?
Have you had this before?

Date
Symptom
Severity
How is this affecting you?
Any ideas what might have caused it?
How are you treating it?
Did you speak to a medical professional or pharmacist and what was the outcome?
Have you had this before?

Date
Symptom
Severity
How is this affecting you?
Any ideas what might have caused it?
How are you treating it?
Did you speak to a medical professional or pharmacist and what was the outcome?
Have you had this before?

Date
Symptom
Severity
How is this affecting you?
Any ideas what might have caused it?
How are you treating it?
Did you speak to a medical professional or pharmacist and what was the outcome?
Have you had this before?

Date
Symptom
Severity
How is this affecting you?
Any ideas what might have caused it?
How are you treating it?
Did you speak to a medical professional or pharmacist and what was the outcome?
Have you had this before?

Date
Symptom
Severity
How is this affecting you?
Any ideas what might have caused it?
How are you treating it?
Did you speak to a medical professional or pharmacist and what was the outcome?
Have you had this before?

Date
Symptom
Severity
How is this affecting you?
Any ideas what might have caused it?
How are you treating it?
Did you speak to a medical professional or pharmacist and what was the outcome?
Have you had this before?

Date
Symptom
Severity
How is this affecting you?
Any ideas what might have caused it?
How are you treating it?
Did you speak to a medical professional or pharmacist and what was the outcome?
Have you had this before?

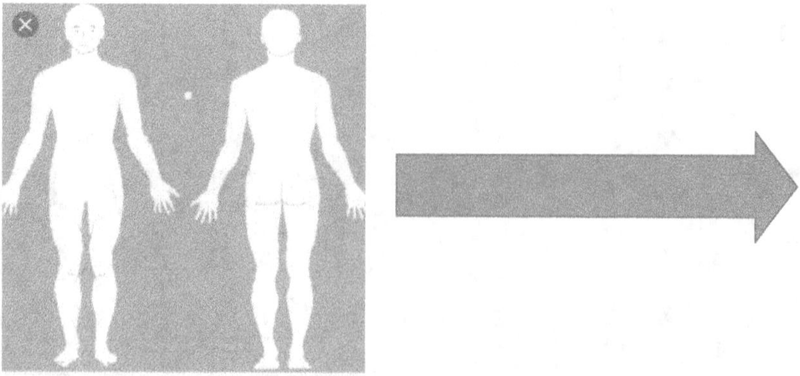

Date
Symptom
Severity
How is this affecting you?
Any ideas what might have caused it?
How are you treating it?
Did you speak to a medical professional or pharmacist and what was the outcome?
Have you had this before?

Date
Symptom
Severity
How is this affecting you?
Any ideas what might have caused it?
How are you treating it?
Did you speak to a medical professional or pharmacist and what was the outcome?
Have you had this before?

8 LIFESTYLE

Which lifestyle changes have you tried, and how well have they worked? What limitations are you currently suffering?

FOOD

ALCOHOL/SMOKING

EXERCISE

ALCOHOL/SMOKING

STRESS

PAIN RELIEF

STRESS

MOBILITY

Inside the house

Outside the house

AIDS AND ADAPTATIONS

To help you bathe

To help you prepare food

To help you dress

To help you sleep

To help you work

OTHER

9 APPOINTMENTS AND REFERRALS

This section is for you to record all the interactions you have with medical professionals, so you can keep track of the questions they asked and the conclusions they drew.

Date
Name of medical professional
Address
Contact number
Speciality
What did you go to them with?
Was it about an existing chronic health condition, or something new?
What questions did they ask, and how did you reply?
What tests did they run?

What conclusions did they draw?

Further treatment?

Further referrals?

Will you need to make an appointment to see them again?

Date
Name of medical professional
Address
Contact number
Speciality
What did you go to them with?
Was it about an existing chronic health condition, or something new?
What questions did they ask, and how did you reply?
What tests did they run?
What conclusions did they draw?

Further treatment?

Further referrals?

Will you need to make an appointment to see them again?

Date
Name of medical professional
Address
Contact number
Speciality
What did you go to them with?
Was it about an existing chronic health condition, or something new?
What questions did they ask, and how did you reply?
What tests did they run?
What conclusions did they draw?

Further treatment?

Further referrals?

Will you need to make an appointment to see them again?

Date
Name of medical professional
Address
Contact number
Speciality
What did you go to them with?
Was it about an existing chronic health condition, or something new?
What questions did they ask, and how did you reply?
What tests did they run?
What conclusions did they draw?

Further treatment?

Further referrals?

Will you need to make an appointment to see them again?

Date
Name of medical professional
Address
Contact number
Speciality
What did you go to them with?
Was it about an existing chronic health condition, or something new?
What questions did they ask, and how did you reply?
What tests did they run?
What conclusions did they draw?

Further treatment?

Further referrals?

Will you need to make an appointment to see them again?

Date
Name of medical professional
Address
Contact number
Speciality
What did you go to them with?
Was it about an existing chronic health condition, or something new?
What questions did they ask, and how did you reply?
What tests did they run?
What conclusions did they draw?

Further treatment?

86

Further referrals?

Will you need to make an appointment to see them again?

Date
Name of medical professional
Address
Contact number
Speciality
What did you go to them with?
Was it about an existing chronic health condition, or something new?
What questions did they ask, and how did you reply?
What tests did they run?
What conclusions did they draw?

<table>
<tr><td>Further treatment?

</td></tr>
<tr><td>Further referrals?

</td></tr>
<tr><td>Will you need to make an appointment to see them again?

</td></tr>
</table>

Date
Name of medical professional
Address
Contact number
Speciality
What did you go to them with?
Was it about an existing chronic health condition, or something new?
What questions did they ask, and how did you reply?
What tests did they run?
What conclusions did they draw?

Further treatment?

Further referrals?

Will you need to make an appointment to see them again?

Date
Name of medical professional
Address
Contact number
Speciality
What did you go to them with?
Was it about an existing chronic health condition, or something new?
What questions did they ask, and how did you reply?
What tests did they run?
What conclusions did they draw?

Further treatment?

Further referrals?

Will you need to make an appointment to see them again?

Date
Name of medical professional
Address
Contact number
Speciality
What did you go to them with?
Was it about an existing chronic health condition, or something new?
What questions did they ask, and how did you reply?
What tests did they run?
What conclusions did they draw?

Further treatment?

Further referrals?

Will you need to make an appointment to see them again?

Date
Name of medical professional
Address
Contact number
Speciality
What did you go to them with?
Was it about an existing chronic health condition, or something new?
What questions did they ask, and how did you reply?
What tests did they run?
What conclusions did they draw?

<table>
<tr><td>Further treatment?

</td></tr>
<tr><td>Further referrals?

</td></tr>
<tr><td>Will you need to make an appointment to see them again?

</td></tr>
</table>

Date
Name of medical professional
Address
Contact number
Speciality
What did you go to them with?
Was it about an existing chronic health condition, or something new?
What questions did they ask, and how did you reply?
What tests did they run?
What conclusions did they draw?

Further treatment?

Further referrals?

Will you need to make an appointment to see them again?

Date
Name of medical professional
Address
Contact number
Speciality
What did you go to them with?
Was it about an existing chronic health condition, or something new?
What questions did they ask, and how did you reply?
What tests did they run?
What conclusions did they draw?

Further treatment?

Further referrals?

Will you need to make an appointment to see them again?

Date
Name of medical professional
Address
Contact number
Speciality
What did you go to them with?
Was it about an existing chronic health condition, or something new?
What questions did they ask, and how did you reply?
What tests did they run?
What conclusions did they draw?

Further treatment?

102

Further referrals?

Will you need to make an appointment to see them again?

Date
Name of medical professional
Address
Contact number
Speciality
What did you go to them with?
Was it about an existing chronic health condition, or something new?
What questions did they ask, and how did you reply?
What tests did they run?
What conclusions did they draw?

Further treatment?

Further referrals?

Will you need to make an appointment to see them again?

Date
Name of medical professional
Address
Contact number
Speciality
What did you go to them with?
Was it about an existing chronic health condition, or something new?
What questions did they ask, and how did you reply?
What tests did they run?
What conclusions did they draw?

Further treatment?

Further referrals?

Will you need to make an appointment to see them again?

Date
Name of medical professional
Address
Contact number
Speciality
What did you go to them with?
Was it about an existing chronic health condition, or something new?
What questions did they ask, and how did you reply?
What tests did they run?
What conclusions did they draw?

<table>
<tr><td>Further treatment?

</td></tr>
<tr><td>Further referrals?

</td></tr>
<tr><td>Will you need to make an appointment to see them again?

</td></tr>
</table>

Date
Name of medical professional
Address
Contact number
Speciality
What did you go to them with?
Was it about an existing chronic health condition, or something new?
What questions did they ask, and how did you reply?
What tests did they run?
What conclusions did they draw?

Further treatment?

Further referrals?

Will you need to make an appointment to see them again?

Date
Name of medical professional
Address
Contact number
Speciality
What did you go to them with?
Was it about an existing chronic health condition, or something new?
What questions did they ask, and how did you reply?
What tests did they run?
What conclusions did they draw?

Further treatment?

Further referrals?

Will you need to make an appointment to see them again?

Date
Name of medical professional
Address
Contact number
Speciality
What did you go to them with?
Was it about an existing chronic health condition, or something new?
What questions did they ask, and how did you reply?
What tests did they run?
What conclusions did they draw?

<table>
<tr><td>Further treatment?

</td></tr>
<tr><td>Further referrals?

</td></tr>
<tr><td>Will you need to make an appointment to see them again?

</td></tr>
</table>

Date
Name of medical professional
Address
Contact number
Speciality
What did you go to them with?
Was it about an existing chronic health condition, or something new?
What questions did they ask, and how did you reply?
What tests did they run?
What conclusions did they draw?

Further treatment?

116

Further referrals?

Will you need to make an appointment to see them again?

Date
Name of medical professional
Address
Contact number
Speciality
What did you go to them with?
Was it about an existing chronic health condition, or something new?
What questions did they ask, and how did you reply?
What tests did they run?
What conclusions did they draw?

Further treatment?

Further referrals?

Will you need to make an appointment to see them again?

Date
Name of medical professional
Address
Contact number
Speciality
What did you go to them with?
Was it about an existing chronic health condition, or something new?
What questions did they ask, and how did you reply?
What tests did they run?
What conclusions did they draw?

Further treatment?

Further referrals?

Will you need to make an appointment to see them again?

Date
Name of medical professional
Address
Contact number
Speciality
What did you go to them with?
Was it about an existing chronic health condition, or something new?
What questions did they ask, and how did you reply?
What tests did they run?
What conclusions did they draw?

Further treatment?

122

Further referrals?

Will you need to make an appointment to see them again?

Date
Name of medical professional
Address
Contact number
Speciality
What did you go to them with?
Was it about an existing chronic health condition, or something new?
What questions did they ask, and how did you reply?
What tests did they run?
What conclusions did they draw?

<table>
<tr><td>

Further treatment?

</td></tr>
<tr><td>

Further referrals?

</td></tr>
<tr><td>

Will you need to make an appointment to see them again?

</td></tr>
</table>

127

10 EXERCISE AND PHYSIOTHERAPY

A lot of illnesses can result in loss of mobility; others can be improved by performing certain exercises. This is a place for you to keep track of your exercise routines and how they affect you.

Date
Exercise
Who told you to do this exercise/ where did you find out about it?
Frequency
Which part of your body does this exercise help?
Positive effects:
Negative effects:

Date
Exercise
Who told you to do this exercise/ where did you find out about it?
Frequency
Which part of your body does this exercise help?
Positive effects:
Negative effects:

Date
Exercise
Who told you to do this exercise/ where did you find out about it?
Frequency
Which part of your body does this exercise help?
Positive effects:
Negative effects:

Date
Exercise
Who told you to do this exercise/ where did you find out about it?
Frequency
Which part of your body does this exercise help?
Positive effects:
Negative effects:

Date
Exercise
Who told you to do this exercise/ where did you find out about it?
Frequency
Which part of your body does this exercise help?
Positive effects:
Negative effects:

Date
Exercise
Who told you to do this exercise/ where did you find out about it?
Frequency
Which part of your body does this exercise help?
Positive effects:
Negative effects:

Date
Exercise
Who told you to do this exercise/ where did you find out about it?
Frequency
Which part of your body does this exercise help?
Positive effects:
Negative effects:

Date
Exercise
Who told you to do this exercise/ where did you find out about it?
Frequency
Which part of your body does this exercise help?
Positive effects:
Negative effects:

Date
Exercise
Who told you to do this exercise/ where did you find out about it?
Frequency
Which part of your body does this exercise help?
Positive effects:
Negative effects:

Date
Exercise
Who told you to do this exercise/ where did you find out about it?
Frequency
Which part of your body does this exercise help?
Positive effects:
Negative effects:

Date
Exercise
Who told you to do this exercise/ where did you find out about it?
Frequency
Which part of your body does this exercise help?
Positive effects:
Negative effects:

Date
Exercise
Who told you to do this exercise/ where did you find out about it?
Frequency
Which part of your body does this exercise help?
Positive effects:
Negative effects:

Date
Exercise
Who told you to do this exercise/ where did you find out about it?
Frequency
Which part of your body does this exercise help?
Positive effects:
Negative effects:

11 DAILY DIARY

We found it helpful to record how our symptoms change over time. It's easiest to do this on a chart like the one below.

It doesn't matter if you forget to record these every day – just write the date in when you do.

We like to use a colour code – RED for very bad, ORANGE for "difficult-but-managing", and GREEN for "I'm fine". You might prefer to use numbers (1 is good – 5 is BAD), or happy/sad faces. It's up to you!

Here's an example:

	SYMPTOMS								TRIGGERS					
DATE	Lower back ache	Headache	Joint pain (arms)	Nausea	Difficulty sleeping	Depression	Anxiety	Constipation	Did exercise routine	Low fat/ high fibre diet	No alcohol	Took cocodamol	Overall health (5 is BAD)	NOTES
15/10/18	5					2	2				x	x	5	too sore to exercise
16/10/18	4		3			2	1	3	x	x	x		4	felt better, went to park
17/10/18	3		2										3	back to work
18/10/18	3												2	

When you look back, you will be able to see whether following certain lifestyle changes or taking certain medicines really do help your symptoms.

On the following pages are several tables where you can specify your own symptoms and triggers.

DATE	SYMPTOMS									TRIGGERS								Overall health (5 is BAD)	NOTES

DATE	SYMPTOMS											TRIGGERS									Overall health (5 is BAD)	NOTES

147

DATE	SYMPTOMS										TRIGGERS									Overall health (5 is BAD)	NOTES

DATE	SYMPTOMS											TRIGGERS										Overall health (5 is BAD)	NOTES

DATE	SYMPTOMS											TRIGGERS							Overall health (5 is BAD)	NOTES

DATE	SYMPTOMS	TRIGGERS	Overall health (5 is BAD)	NOTES

DATE	SYMPTOMS											TRIGGERS									Overall health (5 is BAD)	NOTES

DATE	SYMPTOMS										TRIGGERS								Overall health (5 is BAD)	NOTES

DATE	SYMPTOMS										TRIGGERS									Overall health (5 is BAD)	NOTES

DATE	SYMPTOMS										TRIGGERS								Overall health (5 is BAD)	NOTES

12 CONTACT DETAILS

It's useful to have details of all the medical professionals who treated you, in case you need to go back and query something.

Name	Speciality	Contact details	Notes

Name	Speciality	Contact details	Notes

Name	Speciality	Contact details	Notes

Name	Speciality	Contact details	Notes

13 PLOTS AND PLANS

This is a space for you to list your experiences, thoughts and ideas about your illness. Has someone suggested something which you need to research? Have you been meaning to go and see a particular specialist or try a particular diet or exercise?

14 OUTSIDE HELP

Sometimes you can't do everything yourself. This is a place for you to make a note of any support groups, charities or other agencies that you've approached.

Name of organisation
Address and telephone/email/website details
Name of contact (if you have one)
Date of contact
What help did you ask for?
What help was offered?
Did they suggest any actions for you to carry out?
Will you need to contact them again?
Notes

Name of organisation
Address and telephone/email/website details
Name of contact (if you have one)
Date of contact
What help did you ask for?
What help was offered?
Did they suggest any actions for you to carry out?
Will you need to contact them again?
Notes

Name of organisation
Address and telephone/email/website details
Name of contact (if you have one)
Date of contact
What help did you ask for?
What help was offered?
Did they suggest any actions for you to carry out?
Will you need to contact them again?
Notes

Name of organisation
Address and telephone/email/website details
Name of contact (if you have one)
Date of contact
What help did you ask for?
What help was offered?
Did they suggest any actions for you to carry out?
Will you need to contact them again?
Notes

Name of organisation
Address and telephone/email/website details
Name of contact (if you have one)
Date of contact
What help did you ask for?
What help was offered?
Did they suggest any actions for you to carry out?
Will you need to contact them again?
Notes

15   BENEFITS

It may be helpful to keep a note of the benefits you have applied for and claimed.

Name of benefit
Web link to benefit notes
Date claimed
Claim number
Contact details of claims office
Contact details of anyone who helps you with your claim
Was your claim successful? If not, what happened and is there an appeals process?
Amount awarded:
Date paid from:
Notes (Do you need to do anything to maintain this benefit?)

Name of benefit
Web link to benefit notes
Date claimed
Claim number
Contact details of claims office
Contact details of anyone who helps you with your claim
Was your claim successful? If not, what happened and is there an appeals process?
Amount awarded:
Date paid from:
Notes (Do you need to do anything to maintain this benefit?)

Name of benefit
Web link to benefit notes
Date claimed
Claim number
Contact details of claims office
Contact details of anyone who helps you with your claim
Was your claim successful? If not, what happened and is there an appeals process?
Amount awarded:
Date paid from:
Notes (Do you need to do anything to maintain this benefit?)

Name of benefit
Web link to benefit notes
Date claimed
Claim number
Contact details of claims office
Contact details of anyone who helps you with your claim
Was your claim successful? If not, what happened and is there an appeals process?
Amount awarded:
Date paid from:
Notes (Do you need to do anything to maintain this benefit?)

Name of benefit
Web link to benefit notes
Date claimed
Claim number
Contact details of claims office
Contact details of anyone who helps you with your claim
Was your claim successful? If not, what happened and is there an appeals process?
Amount awarded:
Date paid from:
Notes (Do you need to do anything to maintain this benefit?)

Name of benefit
Web link to benefit notes
Date claimed
Claim number
Contact details of claims office
Contact details of anyone who helps you with your claim
Was your claim successful? If not, what happened and is there an appeals process?
Amount awarded:
Date paid from:
Notes (Do you need to do anything to maintain this benefit?)

ABOUT THE AUTHORS

Lillith May is a young artist living with Ehlers Danlos Syndrome, a painful   genetic condition . It took six years to get diagnosed through the NHS, during which she frequently felt frustrated and marginalised.

You can see (and buy!) her art at
http://www.instagram.com/ Lilustrations

Bekki is her mother, a project manager and author, who also suffers from a chronic health condition.
You can see her art at
http://www.instagram.com/Lucyluton
and her books and other things at http://www.lucyluton.com

They live in Luton with Harry , Steve, Ronnie and a quantity of cats.

Both of them hope you feel better soon xxx

If you have any thoughts or ideas for how to improve this book, please contact felineutopia@gmail.com

13,16,22,28,39,43,61,64,77,79,81,85,88

www.ingramcontent.com/pod-product-compliance
Lightning Source LLC
Chambersburg PA
CBHW071213240726
48654CB00009B/770